The Essential Fatty Liver Diet Guide Recipes and Tips for Liver Health

Manage and Improve Liver Function with Delicious, Health-Promoting Meals

by Dorothy Spencer, BSN RN

TABLE OF CONTENTS

Introduction

In recent years, the prevalence of fatty liver disease has reached alarming levels, affecting an estimated 25% of adults in the United States. This statistic is not just a number; it represents millions of individuals and families grappling with the challenges of managing a condition that often goes unnoticed until it has progressed significantly. For many, a diagnosis of non-alcoholic fatty liver disease (NAFLD) can feel overwhelming, leaving them with questions about how to navigate their health journey. I remember a patient named Sarah, a vibrant 45-year-old mother of two, who was shocked to learn that her liver was struggling due to her dietary choices. Like many, she felt lost and unsure of how to make the necessary changes to improve her health while still enjoying meals with her family.

Purpose

This book, "The Essential Fatty Liver Diet Guide: Recipes and Tips for Liver Health," is designed to empower you with the knowledge and practical tools needed to manage fatty liver disease through diet. My goal is to provide you with clear, actionable advice that can help you make informed dietary choices, create delicious meals, and ultimately improve your liver health. With my background as a registered nurse specializing in liver health and nutrition, I understand the complexities of this condition and the importance of a supportive approach to dietary changes.

In the chapters that follow, you will discover a comprehensive understanding of fatty liver disease, including its causes, symptoms, and the critical role that diet plays in managing your condition. We will explore the fundamentals of a fatty liver diet, essential foods to include, and a variety of delicious recipes that cater to your health needs without sacrificing flavor. Additionally, you will find practical tips for meal planning, lifestyle modifications, and strategies for overcoming challenges along the way.

By the end of this book, you will be equipped with the tools and confidence to take control of your liver health, transforming your relationship with food and paving the way for a healthier future. Together, we will embark on this journey toward better liver health, one meal at a time.

Chapter 1:
Understanding Fatty
Liver Disease

Did you know that fatty liver disease has become the most common liver disorder in the United States, affecting approximately 25% of adults? This staggering statistic is not just a number; it represents millions of individuals and families grappling with the challenges of managing a condition that often goes unnoticed until it leads to more severe liver complications. For many, a diagnosis of non-alcoholic fatty liver disease (NAFLD) can feel overwhelming, leaving them with questions about how to navigate their health journey.

Take Sarah, for example. At 45, she was a vibrant mother of two who enjoyed cooking for her family. When she learned that her liver was struggling due to her dietary choices, she felt lost and unsure of how to make the necessary changes to improve her health while still enjoying meals with her loved ones. This chapter aims to provide you with a comprehensive understanding of fatty liver disease, its implications, and how it can be managed effectively through dietary choices.

What is Fatty Liver Disease?

Definition and Types Fatty liver disease is characterized by the accumulation of excess fat in liver cells. The liver is a vital organ responsible for various functions, including detoxifying harmful substances, producing bile for digestion, and metabolizing nutrients. When fat makes up more than 5-10% of the liver's weight, it is considered fatty liver disease. There are two primary types:

- *Non-Alcoholic Fatty Liver Disease (NAFLD):* This type occurs in individuals who consume little to no alcohol. It is often associated with obesity, diabetes, and metabolic syndrome. NAFLD can progress to non-alcoholic steatohepatitis (NASH), which involves inflammation and can lead to liver damage.

- *Alcoholic Fatty Liver Disease:* This type is caused by excessive alcohol consumption, leading to fat buildup in the liver. It can also progress to more severe liver conditions, such as alcoholic hepatitis or cirrhosis.

Symptoms and Risk Factors Many individuals with fatty liver disease may not experience noticeable symptoms, especially in the early stages. However, some common symptoms can include:

- Fatigue: A general feeling of tiredness that doesn't improve with rest.

- Abdominal Discomfort or Pain: Some may experience discomfort in the upper right abdomen where the liver is located.

- Unexplained Weight Loss: Sudden weight loss without trying can be a sign of liver issues.

- Elevated Liver Enzymes: Detected through blood tests, elevated liver enzymes can indicate liver inflammation or damage.

Risk factors for developing fatty liver disease include:

- Obesity: Excess body weight, particularly around the abdomen, increases the risk of fat accumulation in the liver.

- Type 2 Diabetes: Insulin resistance associated with diabetes can lead to fat buildup in the liver.

- High Cholesterol or Triglycerides: Elevated levels of these fats in the blood can contribute to fatty liver disease.

- Sedentary Lifestyle: Lack of physical activity can lead to weight gain and increase the risk of liver disease.

- Certain Medications: Some medications can contribute to liver fat accumulation.

Importance of Early Diagnosis Early diagnosis of fatty liver disease is crucial for effective management. If left untreated, it can progress to more severe conditions, such as NASH, cirrhosis, or liver cancer. Regular check-ups and liver function tests can help identify the condition before it advances. If you have risk factors for fatty liver disease, it's essential to discuss your concerns with your healthcare provider and consider regular screenings.

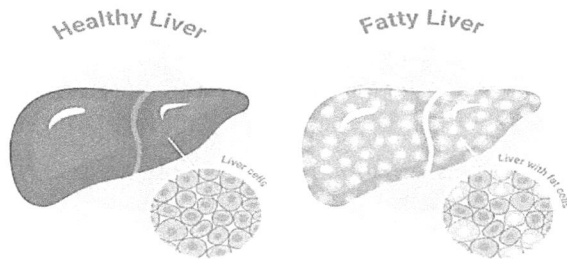

Healthy Liver   Fatty Liver

Liver cells   Liver with fat cells

The Role of Diet in Liver Health

How Diet Affects Liver Function Diet plays a pivotal role in liver health. The liver is responsible for metabolizing nutrients, detoxifying harmful substances, and producing bile for digestion. A diet high in processed foods, sugars, and unhealthy fats can lead to fat accumulation in the liver, exacerbating fatty liver disease. Conversely, a balanced diet rich in whole foods can support liver function and promote overall health.

Key Nutrients for Liver Health Certain nutrients are particularly beneficial for liver health:

- Omega-3 Fatty Acids: Found in fatty fish (like salmon and mackerel), flaxseeds, and walnuts, these healthy fats can help reduce liver fat levels and inflammation. Incorporating omega-3s into your diet can be as simple as enjoying a serving of fish a couple of times a week or adding flaxseed to your smoothies.

- Antioxidants: Vitamins C and E, found in fruits and vegetables, help combat oxidative stress in the liver. Foods like berries, citrus fruits, spinach, and nuts are excellent sources of these vitamins. Including a variety of colorful

6

fruits and vegetables in your meals can enhance your liver's ability to detoxify.

- Fiber: Whole grains, legumes, and vegetables support digestive health and can aid in weight management. Fiber helps regulate blood sugar levels and can assist in reducing fat accumulation in the liver. Aim to include fiber-rich foods in every meal, such as oatmeal for breakfast or a hearty bean salad for lunch.

The Impact of Obesity and Metabolic Syndrome Obesity and metabolic syndrome are significant risk factors for fatty liver disease. Excess body fat, particularly around the abdomen, can lead to insulin resistance and inflammation, further contributing to liver damage. Adopting a balanced diet and maintaining a healthy weight are essential steps in managing and potentially reversing fatty liver disease. Engaging in regular physical activity, such as walking, swimming, or cycling, can also help improve liver health and support weight loss.

Myths and Misconceptions

Common Myths About Fatty Liver Disease

- Myth: **Fatty liver disease only affects heavy drinkers.**

  - Fact: NAFLD can occur in individuals who do not consume alcohol, often linked to obesity and metabolic issues. It's essential to recognize that lifestyle factors, not just alcohol consumption, play a significant role in liver health.

- Myth: **You can't eat fats if you have fatty liver disease.**

  - Fact: Healthy fats, such as those from avocados, nuts, and olive oil, are beneficial for liver health when consumed in moderation. It's important to differentiate between unhealthy trans fats and healthy fats that support overall well-being.

- Myth: **Fatty liver disease is not serious.**

  - Fact: If left untreated, fatty liver disease can lead to severe liver damage and complications. Understanding the potential risks associated with fatty liver disease is crucial for taking proactive steps toward better health.

Clarifying Dietary Misconceptions

Many people are confused about what constitutes a liver-friendly diet. It's essential to focus on whole, nutrient-dense foods rather than eliminating entire food groups. Understanding the difference between healthy and unhealthy fats, as well as the importance of portion control, can empower individuals to make better dietary choices.

Importance of Evidence-Based Information

In a world filled with conflicting dietary advice, it's crucial to rely on evidence-based information. Consulting healthcare professionals and utilizing reputable resources can help individuals navigate their dietary choices effectively. Always seek guidance from registered dietitians or healthcare providers who specialize in liver health to ensure you are making informed decisions.

As we move forward, it's clear that understanding fatty liver disease is just the beginning. The next chapter will focus on the fundamentals of a fatty liver diet, providing you with a structured approach to making dietary changes that can significantly impact your liver health.

Chapter 2: The Basics of a Fatty Liver Diet

Imagine transforming your health simply by changing what's on your plate. The power of diet is profound; it can be the difference between a struggling liver and one that functions optimally. For individuals diagnosed with fatty liver disease, adopting a tailored diet is not just a recommendation—it's a vital step toward reclaiming your health and enhancing your quality of life. In this chapter, we will explore the foundational principles of a fatty liver diet, empowering you to make informed choices that support your liver health.

Key Principles of a Fatty Liver Diet

Focus on Whole Foods vs. Processed Foods

When it comes to managing fatty liver disease, the first principle to embrace is the focus on whole foods. Whole foods are those that are minimally processed and free from artificial ingredients. They include fresh fruits, vegetables, whole grains, lean proteins, and healthy fats. These foods are rich in essential nutrients that support liver function and overall health.

In contrast, processed foods often contain high levels of added sugars, unhealthy fats, and preservatives that can contribute to liver fat accumulation. Examples of processed foods include sugary snacks, fast food, and ready-to-eat meals. By prioritizing whole foods, you can provide your liver with the nutrients it needs to function effectively.

Importance of Balanced Macronutrients

A balanced diet includes an appropriate ratio of macronutrients: carbohydrates, proteins, and fats. Each macronutrient plays a crucial role in your body:

- Carbohydrates: Choose complex carbohydrates, such as whole grains, legumes, and vegetables, which provide sustained energy and fiber. Fiber is particularly important as it aids digestion and helps regulate blood sugar levels.

- Proteins: Incorporate lean protein sources, such as chicken, turkey, fish, beans, and legumes. Protein is essential for repairing tissues and maintaining muscle mass, which can be particularly important if you are working on weight management.

- Fats: Focus on healthy fats, such as those found in avocados, nuts, seeds, and olive oil. These fats can help reduce inflammation and support overall liver health. Avoid trans fats and limit saturated fats, which can contribute to liver fat accumulation.

Staying hydrated is another key principle of a fatty liver diet. Water is essential for various bodily functions, including digestion and detoxification. The liver relies on adequate hydration to effectively process nutrients and eliminate toxins. Aim to drink at least 8-10 cups of water daily, and consider incorporating hydrating foods, such as cucumbers, watermelon, and oranges, into your diet.

As you make these dietary changes, remember to consult with your healthcare provider or a registered dietitian. They can help you tailor your diet to your specific needs and ensure that you are making choices that support your liver health.

Foods to Avoid

High-Sugar Foods and Beverages

One of the most significant contributors to fatty liver disease is excessive sugar intake. Foods and beverages high in added sugars can lead to fat accumulation in the liver. Common culprits include:

- Sugary drinks (sodas, sweetened teas, energy drinks)

- Candy and desserts (cakes, cookies, ice cream)

- Processed snacks (granola bars, flavored yogurts)

Instead of reaching for sugary snacks, opt for fresh fruit or unsweetened yogurt. These alternatives provide natural sweetness along with essential nutrients and fiber.

Saturated and Trans Fats Saturated and trans fats can exacerbate liver fat accumulation and inflammation. Foods high in these unhealthy fats include:

- Fried foods (french fries, fried chicken)

- Processed meats (bacon, sausage, hot dogs)

- Baked goods made with hydrogenated oils (pastries, doughnuts)

To promote liver health, limit your intake of these fats and focus on healthier options, such as cooking with olive oil or enjoying nuts and seeds as snacks.

Alcohol and Its Effects on the Liver

Alcohol consumption can have detrimental effects on liver health, particularly for individuals with fatty liver disease. Alcohol can lead to inflammation, fat accumulation, and liver damage. If you have been diagnosed with fatty liver disease, it is crucial to discuss alcohol consumption with your healthcare provider. They can provide personalized recommendations based on your health status.

Foods to Embrace

Nutrient-Dense Foods (Fruits, Vegetables, Whole Grains)

Incorporating a variety of nutrient-dense foods into your diet is essential for supporting liver health. Focus on:

- Fruits: Berries, apples, oranges, and bananas are excellent choices. They are rich in vitamins, minerals, and antioxidants that help combat oxidative stress in the liver.

- Vegetables: Leafy greens (spinach, kale), cruciferous vegetables (broccoli, cauliflower), and colorful vegetables (bell peppers, carrots) provide essential nutrients and fiber.

- Whole Grains: Choose whole grains like brown rice, quinoa, and whole wheat bread. These grains are high in fiber and can help regulate blood sugar levels.

Lean Proteins and Healthy Fats

In addition to fruits and vegetables, include lean proteins and healthy fats in your diet:

- Lean Proteins: Skinless poultry, fish, beans, and legumes are excellent sources of protein that support muscle health and repair.

- Healthy Fats: Incorporate sources of healthy fats, such as avocados, nuts, seeds, and olive oil. These fats can help reduce inflammation and support overall liver function.

Antioxidant-Rich Foods and Their Benefits

Antioxidants play a vital role in protecting the liver from damage. Foods rich in antioxidants include:

- Berries: Blueberries, strawberries, and raspberries are packed with antioxidants that can help reduce inflammation.

- Nuts and Seeds: Almonds, walnuts, and chia seeds are excellent sources of healthy fats and antioxidants.

- Herbs and Spices: Turmeric, garlic, and ginger have anti-inflammatory properties that can benefit liver health.

Incorporating these foods into your meals can help you create a balanced and liver-friendly diet. As you make these changes, remember to consult with your healthcare provider or a registered dietitian to ensure that your dietary choices align with your health goals.

Understanding which foods to include in your diet is crucial for managing fatty liver disease effectively. In the next chapter, we will delve deeper into specific foods to avoid, ensuring you have a comprehensive understanding of how to protect your liver through dietary choices.

Chapter 3: Essential Foods for Fatty Liver Health

Let me tell you about a patient named Mark, a 50-year-old father of three who came to me feeling defeated after being diagnosed with non-alcoholic fatty liver disease (NAFLD). Mark was overwhelmed by the dietary changes he needed to make and worried about how to provide healthy meals for his family without sacrificing flavor. After working together to develop a tailored meal plan focused on nutrient-dense foods, Mark began to see remarkable changes. Within just a few months, he lost weight, improved his liver function tests, and felt more energetic than he had in years. Mark's journey is a testament to the transformative power of diet, and in this chapter, we will explore the essential foods that can help you achieve similar results.

Comprehensive Food List

To effectively manage fatty liver disease, it's important to understand which foods to include in your diet. Here's a comprehensive list categorized by food groups:

- Fruits:

    - Berries (blueberries, strawberries, raspberries): High in antioxidants and fiber.

    - Apples: Rich in pectin, which helps detoxify the liver.

    - Citrus fruits (oranges, grapefruits, lemons): High in vitamin C and antioxidants.

    - Bananas: Provide potassium and are easy to digest.

- Vegetables:

    - Leafy greens (spinach, kale, Swiss chard): Packed with vitamins and minerals.

    - Cruciferous vegetables (broccoli, cauliflower, Brussels sprouts): Help detoxify the liver.

    - Carrots: High in beta-carotene, which supports liver health.

    - Beets: Contain antioxidants and help improve liver function.

- Proteins:

  - Lean meats (chicken, turkey): Provide essential amino acids without excess fat.

  - Fish (salmon, mackerel, sardines): Rich in omega-3 fatty acids, which reduce liver fat.

  - Legumes (lentils, chickpeas, black beans): High in protein and fiber, promoting satiety.

  - Tofu and tempeh: Plant-based protein sources that are low in fat.

- Grains:

  - Whole grains (brown rice, quinoa, barley): High in fiber and nutrients.

  - Oats: A great source of soluble fiber, which helps lower cholesterol.

  - Whole grain bread and pasta: Opt for varieties made with whole grains for added fiber.

Seasonal and Local Food Options

Eating seasonal and local foods not only supports your health but also benefits the environment. Here are some examples of seasonal foods:

- Spring: Asparagus, peas, strawberries, and radishes.

- Summer: Tomatoes, zucchini, bell peppers, and berries.

- Fall: Pumpkins, sweet potatoes, apples, and kale.

- Winter: Citrus fruits, root vegetables (carrots, turnips), and leafy greens (collard greens, spinach).

Shopping at local farmers' markets can provide you with fresh, high-quality ingredients while supporting local agriculture. Look for organic options when possible, as they are often free from harmful pesticides and chemicals.

Tips for Selecting High-Quality Ingredients

When shopping for groceries, consider the following tips to ensure you select the best ingredients for your liver health:

- Choose Fresh Produce: Look for vibrant colors and firm textures. Avoid fruits and vegetables with bruises or blemishes.

- Read Labels: For packaged foods, check the ingredient list for added sugars, unhealthy fats, and preservatives. Aim for products with minimal ingredients.

- Opt for Grass-Fed and Wild-Caught: When purchasing meat and fish, choose grass-fed beef and wild-caught fish for higher omega-3 content and fewer harmful additives.

- Buy Whole Grains: Look for products labeled "100% whole grain" to ensure you're getting the full nutritional benefits.

Superfoods for Liver Health

Highlight Specific Foods

Certain foods are particularly beneficial for liver health, often referred to as "superfoods." Here are some key superfoods to incorporate into your diet:

- Avocados: Rich in healthy fats and antioxidants, avocados can help reduce liver fat levels. They are also high in fiber, which supports digestion. Try adding sliced avocado to salads or blending it into smoothies for a creamy texture.

- Leafy Greens: Spinach, kale, and Swiss chard are packed with vitamins A, C, and K, as well as antioxidants. These greens help detoxify the liver and reduce fat accumulation. Incorporate them into salads, smoothies, or sauté them as a side dish.

- Nuts: Almonds, walnuts, and pistachios are excellent sources of healthy fats, protein, and fiber. They contain vitamin E, which has been shown to improve liver health. Snack on a handful of nuts or add them to oatmeal or yogurt for added crunch.

- Turmeric: This vibrant yellow spice contains curcumin, a powerful anti-inflammatory compound that can help protect the liver. Use turmeric in curries, soups, or golden milk for a delicious and health-promoting beverage.

- Garlic: Garlic contains sulfur compounds that help detoxify the liver and improve its function. Add minced garlic to stir-fries, roasted vegetables, or salad dressings for flavor and health benefits.

Recipes Featuring These Superfoods

Here are a couple of simple recipes that highlight these superfoods:

- **Avocado and Spinach Smoothie**

    - Ingredients: 1 ripe avocado, 1 cup fresh spinach, 1 banana, 1 cup almond milk, and a tablespoon of honey (optional).

    - Instructions: Blend all ingredients until smooth. Enjoy as a nutritious breakfast or snack.

- **Turmeric Garlic Roasted Vegetables**

    - Ingredients: 2 cups mixed vegetables (carrots, broccoli, bell peppers), 2 tablespoons olive oil, 1 teaspoon turmeric, 2 cloves minced garlic, salt, and pepper to taste.

    - Instructions: Preheat the oven to 400°F (200°C). Toss the vegetables with olive oil, turmeric, garlic, salt, and pepper. Spread on a baking sheet and roast for 20-25 minutes until tender.

Meal Prep Essentials

Importance of Meal Prepping for Success

Meal prepping is a powerful strategy for managing your diet and ensuring you have healthy options readily available. By preparing meals in advance, you can save time, reduce stress, and make healthier choices throughout the week. Here are some benefits of meal prepping:

- Saves Time: Preparing meals in bulk allows you to spend less time cooking during the week. For example, you can cook a large batch of quinoa or brown rice and use it in various meals throughout the week.

- Reduces Food Waste: Planning meals helps you use ingredients efficiently, minimizing waste. If you buy a bunch of spinach, for instance, you can use it in salads, smoothies, and cooked dishes.

- Promotes Healthy Choices: Having healthy meals on hand makes it easier to resist the temptation of unhealthy snacks or takeout. When you're hungry and pressed for time, it's easy to reach for convenience foods, but meal prepping helps you avoid that pitfall.

Tools and Equipment for Efficient Meal Prep

To make meal prepping easier, consider investing in the following tools:

- Food Storage Containers: Use glass or BPA-free plastic containers to store prepped meals. Look for containers with compartments to keep different food items separate. For example, you might have a container with grilled chicken in one section and roasted vegetables in another.

- Meal Prep Containers: Consider using portion-controlled containers to help manage serving sizes. These can be especially helpful for lunches, ensuring you have balanced meals ready to go.

- Sharp Knives and Cutting Boards: Having the right tools makes chopping and preparing ingredients quicker and more efficient. A good chef's knife can make a world of difference when it comes to meal prep.

- Slow Cooker or Instant Pot: These appliances can save time and effort when cooking large batches of meals. For instance, you can throw in a mix of beans, vegetables, and spices in a slow cooker for a hearty chili that cooks while you're busy with other tasks.

Tips for Storing and Reheating Meals

To ensure your prepped meals stay fresh and safe to eat, follow these tips:

- Label Containers: Write the date and contents on each container to keep track of freshness. This way, you can easily see what you have and when it needs to be eaten.

- Store in the Refrigerator or Freezer: Keep meals in the refrigerator for up to four days. For longer storage, freeze meals in airtight containers. For example, you can freeze individual portions of soups or stews for quick meals later.

- Reheat Safely: When reheating meals, ensure they reach an internal temperature of 165°F (74°C) to kill any harmful bacteria. Use the microwave, oven, or stovetop for even heating. If using a microwave, stir the food halfway through to ensure even heating.

- Plan for Variety: To keep meals interesting, plan to use the same ingredients in different ways. For example, if you roast a batch of sweet potatoes, you can use them in a salad, as a side dish, or blended into a soup.

Understanding the essential foods for liver health is a crucial step in your journey toward managing fatty liver disease. In the next chapter, we will explore delicious recipes that incorporate these foods, making it easier for you to enjoy meals that support your health while tantalizing your taste buds.

Chapter 4: Delicious Recipes for Fatty Liver Health

Imagine waking up to the enticing aroma of a warm, spiced oatmeal bowl topped with fresh berries, a drizzle of honey, and a sprinkle of nuts. This delightful breakfast not only satisfies your taste buds but also nourishes your liver, setting a positive tone for the day ahead. In this chapter, we will explore a variety of delicious recipes that are not only healthy but also easy to prepare, ensuring that you and your family can enjoy meals that support liver health without sacrificing flavor.

Breakfast Recipes

Healthy Options Breakfast is often referred to as the most important meal of the day, and for good reason. A nutritious breakfast can kickstart your metabolism and provide the energy you need to tackle the day. Here are some healthy breakfast options:

Berry and Spinach Smoothie

Ingredients

- 1 cup fresh spinach
- 1 cup mixed berries (blueberries, strawberries)
- 1 banana
- 1 cup unsweetened almond milk
- 1 tablespoon chia seeds

Instructions:

- In a blender, combine spinach, mixed berries, banana, almond milk, and chia seeds.
- Blend until smooth and creamy.
- Pour into a glass and enjoy immediately.

Servings: 1

Nutrition Facts (approximate):

- Calories: 250
- Carbohydrates: 45g
- Protein: 6g
- Fats: 7g
- Sodium: 150mg
- Potassium: 600mg
- Fiber: 10g

Why is this recipe good for your liver diet?

This smoothie is packed with antioxidants from the berries and fiber from the spinach and chia seeds, which help reduce inflammation and support liver detoxification. The healthy fats from chia seeds also promote satiety.

Overnight Oats

Ingredients

- 1/2 cup rolled oats
- 1 cup unsweetened almond milk
- 1 tablespoon chia seeds
- 1 tablespoon honey or maple syrup
- Toppings: sliced banana, berries, nuts

Instructions:

- In a jar, combine rolled oats, almond milk, chia seeds, and sweetener.
- Stir well, cover, and refrigerate overnight.
- In the morning, add your favorite toppings and enjoy.

Servings: 1

Nutrition Facts (approximate):

- Calories: 300
- Carbohydrates: 50g
- Protein: 8g
- Fats: 9g
- Sodium: 120mg
- Potassium: 450mg
- Fiber: 12g

Why is this recipe good for your liver diet?

Overnight oats are a great source of soluble fiber, which helps lower cholesterol and supports digestive health. The combination of oats and chia seeds provides sustained energy and keeps you feeling full longer.

Quick and Easy Recipes for Busy Mornings

For those hectic mornings when time is limited, here are some quick and easy breakfast ideas:

- **Greek Yogurt Parfait:**

  Layer Greek yogurt with fresh fruit and a sprinkle of granola for a satisfying breakfast that takes just minutes to prepare.

- **Avocado Toast:**

  Mash half an avocado on whole-grain toast, sprinkle with salt, pepper, and a squeeze of lemon juice. Top with sliced tomatoes or a poached egg for added protein.

- **Chia Seed Pudding**:

  Mix 1/4 cup chia seeds with 1 cup almond milk and a sweetener of your choice. Let it sit for at least 30 minutes or overnight until it thickens. Top with fruit before serving.

- *Experiment with Flavors*: Don't be afraid to try new fruits, spices, or toppings. For example, add cinnamon to your oatmeal or a splash of vanilla extract to your smoothie.

- *Make It Colorful*: A visually appealing breakfast can enhance your enjoyment. Use a variety of colorful fruits and vegetables to make your plate pop.

- *Involve the Family*: Get your family involved in breakfast preparation. Let kids choose their toppings or help with simple tasks like mixing ingredients.

Lunch and Dinner Recipes

Balanced Meals Featuring Lean Proteins and Vegetables

Lunch and dinner are great opportunities to create balanced meals that support liver health. Here are some flavorful recipes:

Quinoa Salad with Grilled Chicken

Ingredients:

- 1 cup cooked quinoa
- 1 grilled chicken breast (sliced)
- 1 cup mixed greens
- 1/2 cup cherry tomatoes (halved)
- 1/4 cucumber (sliced)
- 2 tablespoons olive oil
- Juice of 1 lemon
- Salt and pepper to taste

Instructions:

- In a large bowl, combine cooked quinoa, sliced chicken, mixed greens, cherry tomatoes, and cucumber.
- In a small bowl, whisk together olive oil, lemon juice, salt, and pepper.
- Drizzle the dressing over the salad and toss to combine. Serve immediately.

Servings: 2

Nutrition Facts (approximate per serving):

- Calories: 400

- Carbohydrates: 30g

- Protein: 30g

- Fats: 20g

- Sodium: 200mg

- Potassium: 600mg

- Fiber: 5g

Why is this recipe good for your liver diet?

This salad is rich in lean protein from the chicken and fiber from the quinoa and vegetables, which helps support liver function. The healthy fats from olive oil provide anti-inflammatory benefits.

Baked Salmon with Asparagus

Ingredients List:

- 2 salmon fillets
- 1 bunch asparagus
- 2 tablespoons olive oil
- 2 cloves garlic (minced)
- Salt and pepper to taste
- Lemon wedges for serving

Instructions:

- Preheat the oven to 400°F (200°C).
- Place salmon and asparagus on a baking sheet.
- Drizzle with olive oil, sprinkle with minced garlic, salt, and pepper.
- Bake for 15-20 minutes until the salmon is cooked through and the asparagus is tender.
- Serve with lemon wedges.

Servings: 2

Nutrition Facts (approximate per serving):

- Calories: 350
- Carbohydrates: 8g

- Protein: 30g

- Fats: 22g

- Sodium: 150mg

- Potassium: 800mg

- Fiber: 4g

Why is this recipe good for your liver diet?

Salmon is an excellent source of omega-3 fatty acids, which help reduce liver fat and inflammation. Asparagus is a natural diuretic that supports detoxification, making this dish a liver-friendly option.

Flavorful Dishes That Appeal to the Whole Family

Cooking for the family can be a challenge, but these recipes are sure to please everyone:

- **Vegetable Stir-Fry**: Sauté a mix of colorful vegetables (bell peppers, broccoli, carrots) in a little olive oil with garlic and ginger. Serve over brown rice or quinoa for a quick and nutritious meal.

- **Turkey and Vegetable Chili**: Brown ground turkey in a pot, then add diced tomatoes, kidney beans, black beans, corn, and chili spices. Simmer for 30 minutes for a hearty, flavorful dish.

Cooking Techniques to Enhance Taste Without Added Fats

- **Grilling**: Grilling meats and vegetables can enhance their natural flavors without the need for excessive oils or fats.

- **Roasting**: Roasting vegetables brings out their sweetness. Toss them with herbs and spices before roasting for added flavor.

- **Steaming**: Steaming vegetables preserves their nutrients and natural flavors. Consider steaming broccoli, green beans, or carrots as a side dish.

Snacks and Desserts

Healthy Snack Ideas to Curb Cravings

Snacking can be a healthy part of your diet if you choose the right options. Here are some ideas:

Hummus and Veggies

Ingredients List:

- 1 cup hummus (store-bought or homemade)
- 1 cup assorted raw vegetables (carrot sticks, cucumber slices, bell pepper strips)

Instructions:

- Arrange the raw vegetables on a plate.
- Serve with hummus for dipping.

Servings: 2

Nutrition Facts (approximate per serving):

- Calories: 150
- Carbohydrates: 20g
- Protein: 5g
- Fats: 7g
- Sodium: 200mg
- Potassium: 400mg
- Fiber: 5g

Why is this recipe good for your liver diet?

Hummus is made from chickpeas, which are high in fiber and protein, promoting satiety and digestive health. Pairing it with fresh vegetables adds essential vitamins and minerals while keeping the snack low in calories.

Chia Seed Pudding with Berries

Ingredients List:

- 1/4 cup chia seeds
- 1 cup almond milk
- 1 tablespoon honey or maple syrup
- 1/2 cup fresh berries for topping

Instructions:

- In a bowl, mix chia seeds, almond milk, and sweetener.
- Stir well and let it sit for at least 30 minutes or overnight until it thickens.
- Top with fresh berries before serving.

Servings: 2

Nutrition Facts (approximate per serving):

- Calories: 200
- Carbohydrates: 25g
- Protein: 5g
- Fats: 10g

- Sodium: 50mg

- Potassium: 300mg

- Fiber: 10g

Why is this recipe good for your liver diet?

Chia seeds are rich in omega-3 fatty acids, fiber, and antioxidants, which help reduce inflammation and support liver health. This pudding is a satisfying dessert that is also nutritious.

Quick and Easy Snack Ideas

- **Apple Slices with Almond Butter**:

  Slice an apple and spread a thin layer of almond butter for a delicious combination of sweetness and healthy fats.

- **Popcorn**:

  Air-popped popcorn is a whole grain snack that can be enjoyed plain or seasoned with herbs and spices for flavor.

- **Frozen Banana Bites**

  - Ingredients: 2 ripe bananas, 1/4 cup dark chocolate chips, and chopped nuts (optional).

  - Instructions: Slice bananas into rounds. Melt chocolate chips in a microwave-safe bowl. Dip banana slices in chocolate and sprinkle with nuts if desired. Freeze for 1-2 hours before enjoying.

Importance of Portion Control

While healthy snacks and desserts are great, portion control is essential to avoid overeating. Here are some tips:

- Use Smaller Plates: Serving snacks on smaller plates can help control portions and prevent mindless eating.

- Pre-Portion Snacks: Instead of eating directly from a large bag, portion out snacks into small containers or bags for easy grab-and-go options.

- Listen to Your Body: Pay attention to hunger cues and eat mindfully. Stop eating when you feel satisfied, not stuffed.

With these delicious recipes in your arsenal, you're well on your way to enjoying meals that support your liver health. In the next chapter, we will explore meal planning strategies that will help you stay organized and committed to your dietary goals.

Chapter 5: Meal Planning for Success

Did you know that meal planning can save you up to 30% on your grocery bill while also helping you make healthier food choices? According to research, individuals who plan their meals are more likely to stick to their dietary goals and consume a balanced diet. By taking the time to plan your meals, you can not only save money but also ensure that you and your family are eating foods that support liver health. In this chapter, we will explore effective meal planning strategies that will set you up for success on your journey to better liver health.

Creating a Weekly Meal Plan

Step-by-Step Guide to Meal Planning

Creating a weekly meal plan can seem daunting at first, but breaking it down into manageable steps can make the process easier:

- *Set Aside Time*

  Dedicate a specific time each week to plan your meals. This could be on the weekend or a weekday evening when you have a little extra time.

- *Review Your Schedule*

  Look at your calendar for the week ahead. Consider any days when you may be busy or have plans, and plan simpler meals for those days.

- *Choose Recipes*

  Select recipes that align with your dietary goals and preferences. Aim for a mix of breakfast, lunch, dinner, and snacks. Consider incorporating leftovers into your plan to save time.

- *Create a Meal Calendar*

  Write down your meals for each day of the week. This can be done on paper, a whiteboard, or a digital app. Be sure to include any snacks or beverages.

- *Adjust Portions*

  Consider the number of servings you need for each meal. If you have a family, plan for larger portions, or if you're cooking for yourself, consider how you can use leftovers creatively.

Tips for Balancing Meals Throughout the Week

- **Include a Variety of Food Groups**

  Ensure that each meal includes a balance of protein, healthy fats, and carbohydrates. For example, pair grilled chicken (protein) with quinoa (carbohydrate) and steamed broccoli (vegetable).

46

- **Plan for Color**

  Incorporate a variety of colorful fruits and vegetables throughout the week. This not only makes meals visually appealing but also ensures a range of nutrients.

- **Consider Dietary Needs**

  If you or family members have specific dietary restrictions or preferences (e.g., vegetarian, gluten-free), be sure to accommodate these in your meal plan.

Incorporating Family Preferences

- **Involve the Family**

  Get input from family members about their favorite meals and snacks. This can help ensure everyone is excited about the meal plan.

- **Rotate Favorites**

  Create a rotation of favorite meals to keep things interesting. For example, if your family loves tacos, consider different variations (chicken, fish, or vegetarian) throughout the month.

- **Be Flexible**

  Life can be unpredictable, so be prepared to adjust your meal plan as needed. If something comes up, it's okay to swap meals around or have a backup plan.

Grocery Shopping Tips for a Healthy Liver Diet

Grocery shopping is a fundamental aspect of maintaining a healthy diet, especially when managing conditions like non-alcoholic fatty liver disease (NAFLD). A well-planned shopping trip can help you make informed choices, save money, and ensure that you have all the necessary ingredients to prepare nutritious meals. Here are some comprehensive tips to help you create an effective shopping list, shop on a budget, and understand the importance of reading labels.

How to Create a Shopping List

Review Your Meal Plan

The first step in creating a shopping list is to review your meal plan for the week. This plan should include all the meals you intend to prepare, including breakfast, lunch, dinner, and snacks. By listing all the ingredients needed for each recipe, you can ensure that you have everything on hand when it's time to cook.

For example, if your meal plan includes a quinoa salad with grilled chicken, you'll need to list quinoa, chicken breast, mixed greens, cherry tomatoes, cucumber, and any dressing ingredients. This step not only helps you remember what you need but also minimizes the chances of impulse purchases at the store.

Organize by Category

Once you have your list of ingredients, the next step is to organize them by category. Grouping items into categories such as fruits, vegetables, proteins, grains, and dairy can make your shopping trip more efficient.

For instance, you might have a section for:

- **Fruits**: *Apples, bananas, berries*
- **Vegetables:** *Spinach, broccoli, bell peppers*
- **Proteins**: *Chicken, fish, beans*
- **Grains:** *Quinoa, brown rice, whole grain bread*

By organizing your list this way, you can navigate the grocery store more quickly and avoid backtracking to pick up forgotten items. This organization also helps you visualize your shopping needs and ensures that you don't overlook any essential ingredients.

Check Your Pantry

Before heading to the store, take a moment to check your pantry and refrigerator for items you may already have. This step is crucial for preventing duplicate purchases and reducing food waste.

For example, if you already have olive oil, spices, or canned beans, there's no need to buy more. Additionally, checking your pantry can help you identify ingredients that you can use in your meal planning, allowing you to create meals that utilize what you already have on hand. This practice not only saves money but also encourages creativity in the kitchen.

Plan Around Sales

One of the most effective strategies for shopping on a budget is to plan your meals around sales. Check your local grocery store's weekly ads for discounts on items you need. Many stores offer promotions on fresh produce, meats, and pantry staples, which can significantly reduce your grocery bill.

For instance, if chicken is on sale, consider incorporating it into multiple meals throughout the week. Similarly, if certain vegetables are discounted, plan to use them in salads, stir-fries, or soups. By aligning your meal plan with sales, you can maximize your savings while still eating healthily.

Buy in Bulk

Purchasing non-perishable items in bulk can also lead to significant savings. Items such as grains, beans, nuts, and seeds are often cheaper when bought in larger quantities. Just be sure to store these items properly to maintain their freshness.

For example, store grains in airtight containers in a cool, dry place to prevent spoilage. Buying in bulk not only saves money but also reduces packaging waste, making it an environmentally friendly choice.

Choose Store Brands

When shopping, consider opting for store-brand products instead of name brands. Store-brand items are often less expensive and can be just as high in quality. Many grocery stores have their own brands that offer a wide range of products, from canned goods to dairy items.

For example, if you're looking for canned tomatoes, compare the price and quality of the store brand with a name brand. You may find that the store brand offers the same taste and nutritional value at a lower price.

Importance of Reading Labels

Check for Added Sugars

When purchasing packaged foods, it's essential to read the ingredient list to identify added sugars. Many processed foods contain hidden sugars that can contribute to liver fat accumulation and other health issues. Look for products with minimal ingredients and no added sugars.

For instance, when selecting yogurt, choose plain varieties without added sugars. You can always add fresh fruit or a drizzle of honey for sweetness without the extra sugar content.

Watch for Unhealthy Fats

Be mindful of unhealthy fats when shopping. Avoid products that contain trans fats and limit saturated fats. Instead, look for healthier options, such as those made with olive oil or avocado oil.

For example, when selecting salad dressings, choose those that use healthy fats and natural ingredients. Reading labels can help you make informed choices that support your liver health.

Pay Attention to Serving Sizes

Understanding serving sizes listed on nutrition labels is crucial for managing your dietary intake. Be mindful of how many servings are in a package and adjust your portion sizes accordingly. This can help you better understand the nutritional content of the food you're purchasing.

For instance, if a snack package contains multiple servings, be aware of how many calories, fats, and sugars you're consuming if you eat the entire package. This awareness can help you make healthier choices and maintain portion control.

By following these grocery shopping tips, you can create a well-organized shopping list, shop on a budget, and make informed choices that support your liver health. Remember, the goal is to empower yourself with knowledge and strategies that make healthy eating easier and more enjoyable. With careful planning and mindful shopping, you can set yourself up for success on your journey to better liver health.

Cooking and Preparation Techniques

Healthy Cooking Methods

Steaming

Steaming vegetables helps retain their nutrients and natural flavors without the need for added fats. Consider steaming broccoli, carrots, or green beans as a side dish.

Grilling

Grilling meats and vegetables can enhance their natural flavors while keeping them low in fat. Try grilling chicken, fish, or bell peppers for a delicious meal.

Baking

Baking is a healthy cooking method that requires little to no added fat. Bake salmon, chicken, or vegetables for a nutritious meal.

Batch Cooking and Freezing Meals

Batch Cooking

Prepare large quantities of meals at once, such as soups, stews, or casseroles. This allows you to have ready-to-eat meals throughout the week.

Freezing Meals

Portion out meals into individual containers and freeze them for later use. This is especially helpful for busy days when you don't have time to cook.

Time-Saving Kitchen Hacks

Pre-Chop Vegetables: Spend some time on the weekend chopping vegetables for the week ahead. Store them in airtight containers in the refrigerator for easy access.

Use a Slow Cooker: A slow cooker can be a lifesaver for busy days. Simply add your ingredients in the morning, and come home to a delicious, ready meal.

One-Pan Meals: Look for recipes that can be made in one pan or sheet pan. This not only saves time on cooking but also makes cleanup easier.

Meal planning is a powerful tool that can help you stay organized and committed to your dietary goals. However, it's important to remember that lifestyle changes extend beyond diet. In the next chapter, we will explore the importance of incorporating physical activity and other healthy habits into your daily routine to support your liver health.

Sample 7-Day Meal Plan for Fatty Liver Health

This 7-day meal plan is designed to provide balanced meals that support liver health while incorporating the principles discussed in Chapter 5. Each day includes breakfast, lunch, dinner, and snacks/desserts, along with approximate daily macros. Remember, this is just a sample plan; feel free to adjust it based on your preferences and dietary needs.

Day 1

- Breakfast: Berry and Spinach Smoothie

- Lunch: Quinoa Salad with Grilled Chicken

- Dinner: Baked Salmon with Asparagus

- Snacks: Hummus and Veggies

Daily Macros:

- Calories: 1,300

- Carbohydrates: 150g

- Protein: 80g

- Fats: 50g

- Sodium: 600mg

- Potassium: 1,800mg

- Fiber: 25g

Day 2

- Breakfast: Overnight Oats with Banana and Almonds

- Lunch: Vegetable Stir-Fry with Tofu

- Dinner: Grilled Chicken with Sweet Potato and Broccoli

- Snacks: Greek Yogurt with Berries

Daily Macros:

- Calories: 1,350

- Carbohydrates: 160g

- Protein: 85g

- Fats: 45g

- Sodium: 550mg

- Potassium: 1,900mg

- Fiber: 30g

Day 3

- Breakfast: Avocado Toast with Poached Egg

- Lunch: Lentil Soup with Whole Grain Bread

- Dinner: Turkey and Vegetable Chili

- Snacks: Chia Seed Pudding with Fresh Fruit

Daily Macros:

- Calories: 1,400

- Carbohydrates: 140g

- Protein: 90g

- Fats: 55g

- Sodium: 500mg

- Potassium: 1,850mg

- Fiber: 28g

Day 4

- Breakfast: Chia Seed Pudding with Berries

- Lunch: Spinach and Feta Stuffed Chicken Breast with Quinoa

- Dinner: Shrimp Tacos with Cabbage Slaw

- Snacks: Apple Slices with Almond Butter

Daily Macros:

- Calories: 1,350

- Carbohydrates: 145g

- Protein: 85g

- Fats: 50g

- Sodium: 600mg

- Potassium: 1,800mg

- Fiber: 27g

Day 5

- Breakfast: Greek Yogurt Parfait with Granola and Berries

- Lunch: Grilled Vegetable and Hummus Wrap

- Dinner: Baked Cod with Brown Rice and Green Beans

- Snacks: Mixed Nuts

Daily Macros:

- Calories: 1,400

- Carbohydrates: 150g

- Protein: 80g

- Fats: 60g

- Sodium: 550mg

- Potassium: 1,900mg

- Fiber: 25g

Day 6

- Breakfast: Smoothie Bowl with Banana, Spinach, and Toppings

- Lunch: Chickpea Salad with Cucumber and Tomatoes

- Dinner: Grilled Pork Tenderloin with Roasted Brussels Sprouts

- Snacks: Carrot Sticks with Hummus

Daily Macros:

- Calories: 1,350

- Carbohydrates: 140g

- Protein: 85g

- Fats: 50g

- Sodium: 600mg

- Potassium: 1,800mg

- Fiber: 30g

Day 7

- Breakfast: Oatmeal with Chopped Nuts and Dried Fruit

- Lunch: Quinoa and Black Bean Bowl with Avocado

- Dinner: Stuffed Bell Peppers with Ground Turkey and Brown Rice

- Snacks: Dark Chocolate Covered Almonds

Daily Macros:

- Calories: 1,400

- Carbohydrates: 155g

- Protein: 90g

- Fats: 55g

- Sodium: 500mg

- Potassium: 1,850mg

- Fiber: 28g

Approximate Total Macros for the 7-Day Meal Plan

- Total Calories: 9,100

- Total Carbohydrates: 1,045g

- Total Protein: 505g

- Total Fats: 415g

- Total Sodium: 4,450mg

- Total Potassium: 13,100mg

- Total Fiber: 193g

This 7-day meal plan serves as a useful guide to help you incorporate liver-friendly foods into your diet. While it provides a structured approach, feel free to adjust the meals based on your preferences, dietary needs, and seasonal availability of ingredients. Use this plan as inspiration to create your own meal plans that align with the principles discussed in this book. Remember, the key to success is consistency and making choices that support your health and well-being.

Chapter 6: Lifestyle Modifications for Liver Health

Let me share the inspiring story of Lisa, a 48-year-old woman who was diagnosed with non-alcoholic fatty liver disease (NAFLD) after a routine check-up. Initially, Lisa felt overwhelmed and discouraged, believing that her diagnosis meant she would have to live with limitations. However, after attending a nutrition workshop and learning about the importance of lifestyle changes, she decided to take control of her health. Lisa began incorporating regular physical activity into her routine, practicing mindfulness techniques to manage stress, and engaging her family in her journey toward better health. Over the course of a year, Lisa not only improved her liver function tests but also lost weight, gained energy, and felt more empowered than ever. Her story is a testament to the profound impact that lifestyle modifications can have on liver health, and in this chapter, we will explore the key changes you can make to support your liver.

The Importance of Physical Activity

Physical activity is a cornerstone of a healthy lifestyle, playing a vital role in maintaining liver health and overall well-being. For individuals diagnosed with non-alcoholic fatty liver disease (NAFLD) or other liver conditions, incorporating regular exercise can significantly improve liver function, enhance metabolic health, and promote a better quality of life. In this section, we will explore the recommended types of exercise for liver health, how to create a sustainable exercise routine, and the numerous benefits of regular physical activity.

Recommended Types of Exercise for Liver Health

Aerobic Exercise

Aerobic exercise, also known as cardiovascular exercise, includes activities that increase your heart rate and improve blood circulation. Examples of aerobic exercises include walking, jogging, cycling, swimming, and dancing. Engaging in aerobic exercise is crucial for liver health for several reasons:

- *Weight Management*
  Aerobic exercise helps burn calories, making it an effective tool for weight loss and weight maintenance. Maintaining a healthy weight is essential for managing fatty liver disease, as excess body fat can contribute to liver fat accumulation.

- *Improved Cardiovascular Health*
  Regular aerobic activity strengthens the heart and lungs, reducing the risk of cardiovascular diseases. A healthy cardiovascular system is closely linked to liver health, as it

ensures efficient blood flow and nutrient delivery to the liver.

- *Recommended Duration*
  Aim for at least 150 minutes of moderate-intensity aerobic exercise per week. This can be broken down into manageable sessions, such as 30 minutes of brisk walking five days a week.

Strength Training

Incorporating strength training into your exercise routine is equally important for liver health. Strength training involves resistance exercises that help build muscle mass and improve metabolism. Examples include weight lifting, bodyweight exercises (like push-ups and squats), and resistance band workouts. The benefits of strength training include:

- *Increased Muscle Mass*
  Building muscle mass can enhance your resting metabolic rate, meaning you burn more calories even at rest. This is particularly beneficial for individuals looking to manage their weight and reduce liver fat.
- *Improved Insulin Sensitivity*
  Strength training has been shown to improve insulin sensitivity, which is crucial for preventing type 2 diabetes—a condition often associated with fatty liver disease.
- Recommended Frequency Aim for at least two days of strength training per week, targeting all major muscle

groups. This can include exercises for the arms, legs, back, and core.

Flexibility and Balance Exercises

Flexibility and balance exercises, such as yoga and Pilates, are essential for overall fitness and well-being. These activities offer unique benefits for liver health:

- *Enhanced Flexibility*
  Improved flexibility can help prevent injuries and enhance overall physical performance. This is particularly important as you age or if you are new to exercise.
- *Stress Reduction*
  Many flexibility and balance exercises incorporate mindfulness and relaxation techniques, which can help reduce stress levels. Chronic stress can negatively impact liver health, making these practices particularly beneficial.
- Recommended Activities
  Consider incorporating yoga or Pilates into your routine at least once or twice a week. These practices can be adapted to suit all fitness levels and can be done at home or in a class setting.

Creating a Sustainable Exercise Routine

To reap the benefits of physical activity, it's essential to create a sustainable exercise routine that fits your lifestyle. Here are some tips to help you establish and maintain a consistent exercise regimen:

Set Realistic Goals

Start with achievable goals that align with your current fitness level. For example, if you're new to exercise, aim to walk for 20 minutes a day and gradually increase the duration and intensity of your workouts. Setting small, attainable goals can help you build confidence and motivation.

Find Activities You Enjoy

Choose exercises that you genuinely enjoy. Whether it's dancing, hiking, swimming, or playing a sport, finding activities that you look forward to will make it easier to stick to your routine. Experiment with different types of exercise to discover what you love.

Schedule Workouts

Treat your exercise sessions like appointments. Schedule them into your calendar to ensure you prioritize physical activity. Consistency is key, so try to establish a regular workout routine that fits your daily schedule.

Mix It Up

Incorporate a variety of exercises to keep things interesting and prevent boredom. This can also help you work different muscle groups and improve overall fitness. For example, alternate between aerobic activities, strength training, and flexibility exercises throughout the week.

Regular physical activity offers numerous benefits for liver health and overall well-being. Here are some key advantages:

Weight Management

Exercise helps burn calories and maintain a healthy weight, which is crucial for managing fatty liver disease. Regular physical activity can help reduce liver fat and improve liver function, leading· to better overall health.

Improved Insulin Sensitivity

Physical activity enhances insulin sensitivity, reducing the risk of developing type 2 diabetes and improving liver function. This is particularly important for individuals with fatty liver disease, as insulin resistance is a common issue.

Reduced Inflammation

Regular exercise has anti-inflammatory effects, which can help reduce liver inflammation and improve overall liver health. Inflammation is a key factor in the progression of liver diseases, making it essential to incorporate physical activity into your routine.

Stress Management Techniques

The Connection Between Stress and Liver Health

Chronic stress can have a negative impact on liver health. When you experience stress, your body releases hormones like cortisol, which can lead to increased fat accumulation in the liver and contribute to liver disease. Managing stress is essential for maintaining liver health and overall well-being.

Mindfulness and Relaxation Strategies

Incorporating mindfulness and relaxation techniques into your daily routine can help reduce stress levels. Here are some effective strategies:

Meditation

Practicing mindfulness meditation for just a few minutes each day can help calm the mind and reduce stress. Focus on your breath and allow thoughts to come and go without judgment. Meditation can enhance your overall sense of well-being and promote a positive mindset.

Deep Breathing Exercises

Take a few moments each day to practice deep breathing. Inhale deeply through your nose, hold for a few seconds, and exhale slowly through your mouth. This simple technique can help activate the body's relaxation response and reduce feelings of stress and anxiety.

Yoga

Engaging in yoga can promote relaxation, improve flexibility, and reduce stress. Consider joining a local class or following online tutorials. Yoga combines physical movement with mindfulness, making it an excellent practice for both body and mind.

Nature Walks

Spending time in nature can have a calming effect on the mind and body. Take a walk in a park or garden to enjoy the benefits of fresh air and natural surroundings. Nature has been shown to reduce stress levels and improve mood.

Importance of Sleep for Recovery

Adequate sleep is essential for overall health and liver function. During sleep, the body undergoes important processes for recovery and detoxification. Aim for 7-9 hours of quality sleep each night. Here are some tips for improving sleep quality:

Establish a Sleep Routine

Go to bed and wake up at the same time each day to regulate your body's internal clock. Consistency in your sleep schedule can help improve the quality of your sleep.

Create a Relaxing Environment

Make your bedroom a calming space by keeping it dark, quiet, and cool. Consider using blackout curtains and white noise machines if needed. A comfortable sleep environment can significantly enhance your ability to fall asleep and stay asleep.

Limit Screen Time

Reduce exposure to screens (phones, computers, TVs) at least an hour before bedtime, as blue light can interfere with sleep quality. Instead, consider reading a book or practicing relaxation techniques to wind down before sleep.

Incorporating physical activity, stress management techniques, and adequate sleep into your daily routine is essential for maintaining liver health and overall well-being. By understanding the importance of these lifestyle modifications and implementing them into your life, you can take proactive steps toward managing fatty liver disease and improving your quality of life. Remember, every small change counts, and with dedication and commitment, you can achieve your health goals and enjoy a healthier future.

Building a Support System

When it comes to managing liver health, particularly for those diagnosed with conditions like non-alcoholic fatty liver disease (NAFLD), having a strong support system can make a significant difference in your journey. Engaging family and friends, finding support groups, and utilizing healthcare professionals are all essential components of a comprehensive approach to health management. In this section, we will explore how to build a robust support system that can empower you to achieve your health goals.

Engaging Family and Friends in the Journey

Having a strong support system can make a significant difference in your journey toward better liver health. Here are some ways to engage family and friends:

Share Your Goals

The first step in building a support system is to communicate your health goals with family and friends. Sharing your objectives not only helps them understand your journey but also allows them to provide encouragement and support. When your loved ones are aware of your goals—whether it's losing weight, eating healthier, or exercising more—they can help hold you accountable and celebrate your successes along the way.

For example, if you aim to reduce your liver fat through dietary changes, let your family know about the specific foods you want to incorporate into your meals. This way, they can support you by joining you in making healthier choices, whether it's cooking together or choosing restaurants that offer liver-friendly options.

Involve Them in Meal Prep

Cooking can be a fun and rewarding activity, especially when shared with others. Involving family members in meal planning and preparation can strengthen your support system while making healthy choices together. Consider setting aside a day each week for meal prep, where everyone can contribute to creating nutritious meals for the week ahead.

For instance, you might designate Sunday afternoons for meal prep. Gather your family in the kitchen, and assign tasks such as chopping vegetables, marinating proteins, or assembling healthy snacks. Not only does this make the process more enjoyable, but it also fosters a sense of teamwork and shared responsibility for health.

Additionally, cooking together provides an opportunity to educate your family about the importance of liver health and the benefits of a balanced diet. You can share recipes, discuss nutritional information, and even experiment with new ingredients. This collaborative approach can help create a supportive environment where everyone is invested in making healthier choices.

Exercise Together

Physical activity is a crucial component of liver health, and exercising with friends or family can make it more enjoyable and motivating. Encourage your loved ones to join you for workouts, outdoor activities, or even leisurely walks. This not only helps you stay accountable but also strengthens your relationships.

For example, you could organize a weekly family hike or a group workout session at a local gym. If you prefer home workouts, consider following online exercise classes together. The camaraderie of exercising with others can make the experience more enjoyable and less daunting, especially if you're new to fitness.

Moreover, exercising together can provide an opportunity for open discussions about health and wellness. You can share your experiences, challenges, and successes, creating a supportive atmosphere where everyone feels encouraged to pursue their health goals.

Finding Support Groups and Resources

Connecting with others who are on a similar journey can provide valuable support and encouragement. Consider the following options:

Support Groups

Look for local or online support groups focused on liver health or fatty liver disease. These groups can be a source of empowerment, as they allow individuals to share their experiences, challenges, and advice. Being part of a community that understands your struggles can help you feel less isolated and more motivated to make positive changes.

Many hospitals and health organizations offer support groups for individuals with liver conditions. These groups often provide educational resources, guest speakers, and opportunities for networking with others facing similar challenges. If you prefer online options, consider joining forums or social media groups dedicated to liver health. These platforms can provide a sense of community and access to valuable information.

Community Programs

Many communities offer health and wellness programs that focus on nutrition, exercise, and lifestyle changes. Check with local health organizations, community centers, or hospitals for resources that may be available in your area. These programs often include workshops, cooking classes, and fitness sessions designed to promote healthy living.

Participating in community programs can also help you meet like-minded individuals who share your health goals. Building connections with others in these programs can lead to lasting friendships and additional support in your journey toward better liver health.

Online Forums

In today's digital age, online forums and social media groups can be excellent resources for finding support and information. Joining online communities dedicated to liver health allows you to connect with individuals from around the world who are navigating similar challenges. These platforms can provide a wealth of knowledge, from sharing personal experiences to discussing the latest research and dietary tips.

When participating in online forums, remember to engage respectfully and thoughtfully. Share your insights, ask questions, and offer support to others. The sense of community that develops in these spaces can be incredibly uplifting and motivating.

The Role of Healthcare Professionals

Don't hesitate to reach out to healthcare professionals for guidance and support. This may include:

Registered Dietitians

A registered dietitian can help you create a personalized meal plan that aligns with your health goals and dietary needs. They can provide valuable insights into nutrition, helping you understand which foods are best for your liver health and how to incorporate them into your meals. Working with a dietitian can also help you navigate any dietary restrictions or preferences you may have.

During your sessions, be open about your goals, challenges, and any specific concerns you have regarding your diet. A dietitian can offer tailored advice and strategies to help you succeed.

Personal Trainers

If you're unsure where to start with exercise, consider working with a personal trainer who can design a workout plan tailored to your fitness level and goals. A trainer can provide guidance on proper form, help you set realistic fitness goals, and keep you motivated throughout your journey.

When selecting a personal trainer, look for someone with experience in working with individuals who have health conditions or specific fitness goals. This ensures that your workouts are safe and effective.

Healthcare Providers

Regular check-ups with your doctor are essential for monitoring your liver health and providing ongoing support as you make lifestyle changes. Your healthcare provider can help track your progress, adjust your treatment plan as needed, and address any concerns you may have.

During your appointments, be proactive in discussing your health goals and any challenges you're facing. Your doctor can offer valuable insights and resources to help you stay on track.

Building a strong support system is a vital component of managing fatty liver disease and making lasting dietary changes. By engaging family and friends, connecting with support groups, and utilizing healthcare professionals, you can create a network of support that empowers you to achieve your health goals. Remember, you are not alone on this journey, and with the right support, you can navigate the challenges and celebrate your successes as you work toward better liver health.

Making lifestyle modifications is a crucial step in managing fatty liver disease and improving overall health. In the next chapter, we will discuss how to monitor your progress effectively, ensuring that you stay on track and continue to make positive changes.

Chapter 7: Monitoring Your Progress

Did you know that individuals who actively track their health metrics are 50% more likely to achieve their health goals? Monitoring your progress is a crucial component of managing fatty liver disease and making lasting lifestyle changes. By keeping an eye on your health metrics, you can identify trends, celebrate successes, and make informed decisions about your diet and lifestyle. In this chapter, we will explore effective strategies for monitoring your progress, including understanding liver function tests, keeping a food journal, and setting realistic health goals.

Understanding Liver Function Tests

Explanation of Common Liver Function Tests

Liver function tests (LFTs) are blood tests that measure various enzymes, proteins, and substances produced by the liver. These tests help assess the liver's health and function. Common tests include:

- **Alanine Aminotransferase (ALT):** Elevated levels of ALT can indicate liver inflammation or damage.

- **Aspartate Aminotransferase (AST)**: Like ALT, high AST levels can suggest liver issues, but they can also be elevated due to other conditions.

- **Alkaline Phosphatase (ALP):** This enzyme is associated with bile duct function. Elevated levels may indicate bile duct obstruction or liver disease.

- **Bilirubin:** This substance is produced during the breakdown of red blood cells. High bilirubin levels can indicate liver dysfunction or bile duct problems.

- **Albumin**: This protein is produced by the liver. Low levels may suggest liver disease or other health issues.

How to Interpret Results

Understanding your liver function test results is essential for monitoring your liver health. Here's a general guide to interpreting the results:

- **Normal Ranges**: Each lab may have slightly different reference ranges, so it's important to discuss your results with your healthcare provider.

- **Elevated Enzymes:** If your ALT and AST levels are elevated, it may indicate liver inflammation or damage. Your doctor may recommend further testing or lifestyle changes.

- **Bilirubin Levels**: Elevated bilirubin levels may require additional evaluation to determine the underlying cause.

- **Regular Monitoring**: Regular liver function tests can help track changes over time and assess the effectiveness of dietary and lifestyle modifications.

Importance of Regular Check-Ups

Regular check-ups with your healthcare provider are crucial for monitoring liver health. These visits allow for:

- **Early Detection:** Routine testing can help identify liver issues before they progress to more serious conditions.

- **Personalized Guidance**: Your healthcare provider can offer tailored advice based on your test results and overall health.

- **Accountability**: Regular appointments can help keep you motivated and accountable for your health goals.

Keeping a Food Journal

Keeping a food journal is a powerful tool for anyone looking to manage their diet, especially for individuals dealing with conditions like non-alcoholic fatty liver disease (NAFLD). By tracking what you eat, you can gain valuable insights into your dietary habits, identify areas for improvement, and ultimately make more informed choices that support your health. In this section, we will explore the benefits of tracking dietary intake, tips for maintaining a food journal, how to use it for accountability, and the importance of setting realistic goals.

Increased Awareness

One of the most significant benefits of keeping a food journal is the increased awareness it brings to your eating habits. When you write down everything you consume, you become more conscious of your dietary choices. This awareness can help you identify patterns in your eating behavior, such as emotional eating or mindless snacking.

For example, you may notice that you tend to reach for sugary snacks when you're feeling stressed or that you skip meals when you're busy. By recognizing these patterns, you can take proactive steps to address them. Increased awareness can also help you identify areas for improvement, such as incorporating more fruits and vegetables into your diet or reducing your intake of processed foods.

Accountability

A food journal serves as a form of accountability, helping you stay committed to your health goals. When you know that you will be recording your food intake, you may be more mindful of your choices. This accountability can be particularly beneficial when you're tempted to indulge in unhealthy foods.

For instance, if you're trying to reduce your sugar intake, seeing it written down in your journal can serve as a reminder of your commitment to healthier choices. Additionally, sharing your food journal with a trusted friend or family member can further enhance accountability, as they can provide support and encouragement along the way.

Identifying Triggers

Tracking your food intake can also help you identify triggers related to cravings, energy levels, or digestive issues. By noting what you eat and how you feel afterward, you can begin to see connections between your food choices and your physical or emotional state.

For example, if you consistently feel sluggish after consuming certain foods, you may want to reconsider including them in your diet. Similarly, if you notice that specific situations or emotions lead to unhealthy eating patterns, you can develop strategies to cope with those triggers more effectively. This insight can empower you to make healthier choices that align with your goals.

Tips for Maintaining a Food Journal

Choose Your Format

The first step in maintaining a food journal is to choose a format that works best for you. You can opt for a physical notebook, a digital app, or a spreadsheet. Each format has its advantages, so consider what will be most convenient and motivating for you.

- *Physical Notebook*: A traditional notebook allows for creativity and personalization. You can use colored pens, stickers, or drawings to make it visually appealing.
- *Digital Apps*: Many apps are designed specifically for tracking food intake, offering features like barcode scanning, nutritional information, and meal suggestions. Popular options include **MyFitnessPal**, **Lose It**!, and **Cronometer**.

- *Spreadsheet*: If you prefer a more structured approach, using a spreadsheet can help you organize your entries and analyze your data over time.

Be Consistent

Consistency is key to gaining valuable insights into your eating habits. Aim to record your meals and snacks daily, including portion sizes and preparation methods. The more detailed your entries, the more information you'll have to work with when reviewing your progress.

Set a specific time each day to update your food journal, whether it's after each meal or at the end of the day. This routine can help you stay committed and make tracking a habit.

Include Details

When keeping a food journal, it's essential to include not only what you eat but also additional details that can provide context. Note portion sizes, preparation methods (e.g., grilled, baked, fried), and any accompanying feelings (e.g., hungry, satisfied, stressed).

For example, instead of simply writing "salad," you might note "large mixed greens salad with cherry tomatoes, cucumbers, and balsamic vinaigrette." Including these details can help you identify patterns and make more informed choices in the future.

How to Use the Journal for Accountability

Review Regularly

Set aside time each week to review your food journal. Look for patterns, successes, and areas for improvement. This reflection can help you stay accountable to your health goals and make necessary adjustments to your diet.

For instance, if you notice that you consistently struggle with late-night snacking, you can develop strategies to address this behavior, such as preparing healthier snacks in advance or finding alternative activities to engage in during those times.

Share with a Support System

Consider sharing your food journal with a trusted friend, family member, or healthcare provider for additional accountability and support. Having someone else aware of your goals can provide motivation and encouragement, making it easier to stay on track.

You might also consider joining a support group where members share their food journals and experiences. This can foster a sense of community and provide valuable insights from others who are on similar journeys.

Set Goals Based on Insights

Use the information from your journal to set specific dietary goals. For example, if you notice that you're not consuming enough vegetables, you might set a goal to include at least one serving of vegetables in each meal.

Setting clear, actionable goals based on your journal entries can help you stay focused and motivated as you work toward improving your liver health.

Importance of Setting Achievable Health Goals

Setting realistic and achievable health goals is essential for long-term success. Here's why:

- *Motivation*: Achievable goals can boost your motivation and confidence as you see progress. When you set small, attainable goals, you're more likely to experience success, which can encourage you to continue making healthy choices.

- *Focus:* Clear goals help you stay focused on what you want to achieve, making it easier to create a plan of action. For example, if your goal is to increase your vegetable intake, you can plan meals that incorporate a variety of vegetables.

- *Sustainability*: Setting realistic goals ensures that you can maintain your changes over time without feeling overwhelmed. It's important to recognize that lifestyle changes take time, and gradual progress is often more sustainable than drastic changes.

Strategies for Tracking Progress

SMART Goals

Use the SMART criteria to set goals that are Specific, Measurable, Achievable, Relevant, and Time-bound. For example, "I will walk for 30 minutes, five days a week for the next month." This approach helps clarify your goals and makes it easier to track your progress.

Use a Progress Tracker

Consider using a journal, app, or chart to track your progress toward your goals. This can help you visualize your achievements and stay motivated. Seeing your progress over time can reinforce your commitment to your health journey.

Regular Check-Ins

Schedule regular check-ins with yourself to assess your progress and make any necessary adjustments to your goals. This reflection can help you stay accountable and ensure that you're on track to meet your health objectives.

Celebrating Small Victories

Acknowledge Achievements: Take time to celebrate your successes, no matter how small. This could be as simple as treating yourself to a favorite healthy meal or enjoying a relaxing activity. Acknowledging your achievements reinforces positive behavior and motivates you to continue making healthy choices.

Share with Others: Share your victories with friends or family members who support your journey. Their encouragement can help reinforce your commitment to your health. Celebrating together can create a sense of community and shared success.

Reflect on Your Journey: Regularly reflect on how far you've come and the positive changes you've made. This can help you stay motivated and focused on your long-term goals. Consider keeping a section in your food journal dedicated to reflections, where you can write about your experiences, challenges, and successes.

In conclusion, keeping a food journal is a valuable tool for managing your diet and monitoring your progress, especially when dealing with liver health. By increasing awareness of your dietary choices, holding yourself accountable, and identifying triggers, you can make informed decisions that support your health goals. With consistent effort and a commitment to self-reflection, you can create a sustainable approach to healthy eating that empowers you on your journey to better liver health.

Monitoring your progress is a vital part of managing fatty liver disease and making lasting lifestyle changes. In the next chapter, we will discuss how to overcome challenges that may arise on your journey, ensuring that you stay on track and continue to make positive changes.

Chapter 8: Overcoming Challenges in Dietary Changes

Meet Tom, a 55-year-old man who was diagnosed with non-alcoholic fatty liver disease (NAFLD) after years of unhealthy eating habits. Tom was determined to make changes, but he quickly faced challenges that many individuals with fatty liver disease encounter. He struggled with cravings for his favorite comfort foods, felt overwhelmed at social gatherings, and sometimes lost motivation when progress seemed slow. However, with the right strategies and support, Tom learned how to navigate these challenges and stay committed to his health journey. His story is a reminder that while dietary changes can be difficult, they are achievable with the right mindset and tools. In this chapter, we will explore common challenges faced by individuals with fatty liver disease and provide practical strategies for overcoming them.

Managing dietary changes, especially for individuals with conditions like non-alcoholic fatty liver disease (NAFLD), can be a daunting task. Cravings, social situations, and maintaining motivation are just a few of the challenges that can arise. However, with the right strategies and mindset, these challenges can be effectively managed. This section will delve into practical approaches for dealing with cravings and temptations, navigating social situations, and staying motivated throughout your health journey.

Dealing with Cravings and Temptations

Strategies for Managing Cravings

Cravings are a normal part of any dietary change, particularly when you're trying to adopt healthier eating habits. Understanding how to manage these cravings is crucial for long-term success. Here are some effective strategies:

- *Identify Triggers:* The first step in managing cravings is to identify what triggers them. Is it stress, boredom, or certain social situations? Keeping a food journal can help you pinpoint these triggers. For example, if you notice that you crave sweets after a stressful day at work, you can develop alternative coping strategies, such as going for a walk or practicing deep breathing exercises instead of reaching for dessert.
- *Stay Hydrated:* Thirst can often be mistaken for hunger, leading to unnecessary snacking. Make sure you're drinking enough water throughout the day. Aim for at least 8-10 cups of water daily. If you find yourself craving a snack, try drinking a glass of water first and waiting a few minutes to see if the craving subsides.
- *Practice Mindful Eating*: When cravings strike, take a moment to pause and assess whether you're truly hungry.

Mindful eating involves being present during meals, savoring each bite, and listening to your body's hunger cues. This practice can help you differentiate between physical hunger and emotional cravings, allowing you to make more conscious choices.

Healthy Alternatives to Common Cravings

Instead of giving in to unhealthy cravings, consider these healthier alternatives:

- *Sweet Cravings:* If you crave something sweet, opt for fresh fruit, yogurt with honey, or a small piece of dark chocolate. These options provide natural sweetness along with nutrients. For instance, a bowl of mixed berries can satisfy your sweet tooth while offering antioxidants and fiber.
- *Salty Cravings:* For salty snacks, try air-popped popcorn, roasted chickpeas, or a handful of nuts. These alternatives can satisfy your craving without the unhealthy additives found in processed snacks. For example, seasoned roasted chickpeas can provide a crunchy, savory snack that is high in protein and fiber.
- *Comfort Food Cravings*: If you're craving comfort foods like mac and cheese, try making a healthier version using whole grain pasta, low-fat cheese, and added vegetables for extra nutrition. This way, you can enjoy the flavors you love while still making a healthier choice.

Importance of Moderation

While it's important to make healthier choices, it's also essential to allow yourself the occasional treat. Practicing moderation can help prevent feelings of deprivation and make it easier to stick to your dietary changes. Here are some tips:

- *Portion Control*: If you indulge in a favorite treat, keep the portion small. Enjoying a small serving can satisfy your craving without derailing your progress. For example, instead of a large slice of cake, opt for a small piece and savor it.
- *Plan for Treats:* Incorporate occasional treats into your meal plan. Knowing you have a special treat to look forward to can help you stay motivated and committed to your healthy choices. For instance, if you plan to enjoy a dessert at a family gathering, you can adjust your meals earlier in the day to accommodate that treat.

Navigating Social Situations

Social situations can present unique challenges when trying to maintain a healthy diet. Here are some tips for navigating these scenarios:

Tips for Dining Out and Attending Events

Research Menus Ahead of Time

If you're dining out, check the restaurant's menu online before you go. Look for healthier options that align with your dietary goals. Many restaurants now offer nutritional information on their websites, making it easier to make informed choices.

- **Choose Wisely**

Opt for grilled, baked, or steamed dishes rather than fried or creamy options. Don't hesitate to ask for modifications, such as dressing on the side or substituting vegetables for fries. For example, if you're at a restaurant, you might choose a grilled chicken salad with vinaigrette on the side instead of a fried chicken sandwich.

- **Plan Ahead for Events**

  If you're attending a gathering, consider bringing a healthy dish to share. This ensures you have at least one nutritious option available. You could prepare a colorful vegetable platter with hummus or a quinoa salad that everyone can enjoy.

Communicating Dietary Needs to Others

It's important to communicate your dietary needs to friends and family, especially when attending social events. Here are some strategies:

- **Be Open and Honest**

  Share your health goals with those close to you. Most people will be supportive and willing to accommodate your dietary needs. For instance, you might say, "I'm trying to eat healthier for my liver, so I'm focusing on whole foods and reducing sugar."

- **Suggest Alternatives**

  If you're invited to a restaurant or event, suggest places that offer healthier options. This can help ensure you have choices that align with your dietary goals. If a friend suggests a restaurant, you could respond with, "How about we go to that new place that has great salads and grilled options?"

- **Practice Assertiveness**

  Don't be afraid to politely decline foods that don't fit your dietary needs. You can say something like, "I appreciate the offer, but I'm focusing on my health right now." Most people will respect your decision if you communicate it kindly.

Finding Balance in Social Settings

Finding balance in social situations is key to maintaining your dietary changes. Here are some tips:

- **Enjoy the Company**

  Focus on the social aspect of gatherings rather than solely on the food. Engage in conversations and activities to shift your focus away from eating. This can help you enjoy the event without feeling pressured to indulge in unhealthy foods.

- **Practice Mindful Eating**

  If you do indulge, savor each bite and enjoy the flavors. This can help you feel more satisfied and prevent overeating. Take your time to eat slowly and appreciate the meal, rather than rushing through it.

- **Set Boundaries**

  It's okay to set boundaries for yourself. Decide in advance how many treats you'll allow yourself at an event and stick to that decision. For example, you might decide to enjoy one dessert but skip the chips and dip.

Staying motivated on your health journey can be challenging, but there are several techniques that can help:

Techniques for Maintaining Motivation

Visualize Your Goals: Create a vision board or write down your health goals. Visual reminders can help keep you focused and motivated. Include images of healthy foods, activities you enjoy, and quotes that inspire you.

Track Your Progress: Keep a journal or use an app to track your dietary changes, exercise, and any improvements in your health. Seeing your progress can boost your motivation. For example, you might note how you feel after a week of healthy eating or how your energy levels have improved.

Set Short-Term Goals: In addition to long-term goals, set short-term, achievable goals. Celebrate these small victories to maintain motivation. For instance, if your long-term goal is to lose weight, a short-term goal could be to incorporate more vegetables into your meals for the next week.

Importance of Self-Compassion

It's essential to practice self-compassion throughout your journey. Here's how:

Be Kind to Yourself: Understand that setbacks are a normal part of any lifestyle change. Instead of being critical, treat yourself with kindness and focus on getting back on track. If you indulge in a treat, remind yourself that one slip-up doesn't define your journey.

Avoid Perfectionism: Striving for perfection can lead to frustration. Aim for progress rather than perfection, and remember that every healthy choice counts. Celebrate the small changes you make, even if they don't seem significant at first.

Reflect on Your Journey: Take time to reflect on how far you've come. Acknowledge the positive changes you've made and the challenges you've overcome. This reflection can help you stay motivated and focused on your long-term goals.

Seeking Inspiration from Success Stories

Reading or hearing about others' success stories can provide motivation and encouragement. Consider the following:

Join Support Groups: Engage with support groups, either in-person or online, where members share their experiences and successes. This can provide a sense of community and inspiration. Hearing how others have overcome challenges can motivate you to stay committed to your goals.

Follow Health Influencers: Look for health and wellness influencers who focus on liver health or healthy eating. Their stories and tips can offer valuable insights and motivation. Many influencers share their personal journeys, including struggles and triumphs, which can resonate with your own experiences.

Share Your Story: As you progress on your journey, consider sharing your own story. This can inspire others and reinforce your commitment to your health goals. Whether through social media, a blog, or a support group, sharing your experiences can create a sense of connection and accountability.

Overcoming challenges in dietary changes is an essential part of managing fatty liver disease and making lasting lifestyle changes. By implementing strategies for managing cravings, navigating social situations, and staying motivated, you can create a supportive environment that fosters your health journey. Remember, it's normal to face obstacles along the way, but with determination and the right support, you can achieve your health goals and enjoy a healthier, more fulfilling life.

Chapter 9: The Future of Liver Health

"Health is not just about what you're eating. It's also about what you're thinking and saying." – Louise Hay. This quote beautifully encapsulates the holistic approach needed for optimal health and wellness, especially when it comes to managing liver health. As we look toward the future, it's essential to embrace not only dietary changes but also a mindset that fosters continuous learning and community support. In this chapter, we will explore emerging research in liver health, the importance of community engagement, and the value of lifelong learning and adaptation.

Emerging Research in Liver Health

The field of liver health is rapidly evolving, with ongoing research aimed at understanding the complexities of liver diseases, including non-alcoholic fatty liver disease (NAFLD) and its progression. As our understanding of liver health deepens, several key research trends have emerged that highlight the intricate relationships between diet, genetics, and overall health. This section will explore these trends, innovations in dietary approaches, and the role of technology in health monitoring.

Gut-Liver Axis

One of the most exciting areas of research in liver health is the exploration of the gut-liver axis. This concept refers to the bidirectional relationship between the gut microbiome and liver function. Researchers are investigating how the composition of gut bacteria can influence liver health and vice versa.

Studies suggest that a healthy gut microbiome may play a role in preventing liver diseases and improving liver function. For example, a study published in the journal *Hepatology* found that individuals with NAFLD often have an altered gut microbiome, characterized by a decrease in beneficial bacteria and an increase in harmful bacteria. This imbalance can lead to increased intestinal permeability, allowing toxins to enter the bloodstream and contribute to liver inflammation.

Furthermore, dietary interventions that promote a healthy gut microbiome, such as increasing fiber intake and consuming fermented foods, are being studied for their potential to improve liver health. Foods rich in probiotics, like yogurt and kefir, and prebiotics, such as garlic and onions, may help restore balance to the gut microbiome and support liver function.

Nutritional Interventions

There is a growing body of evidence supporting the role of specific dietary interventions in managing liver health. Research is focusing on the benefits of Mediterranean diets, plant-based diets, and the impact of specific nutrients on liver function.

The Mediterranean diet, which emphasizes whole grains, fruits, vegetables, healthy fats (like olive oil), and lean proteins (such as fish and poultry), has been shown to have protective effects on liver health. A study published in *The American Journal of Clinical Nutrition* found that adherence to a Mediterranean diet was associated with a lower risk of developing NAFLD.

Similarly, *plant-based diets* are gaining attention for their potential benefits in reducing liver fat and inflammation. Research indicates that diets rich in fruits, vegetables, whole grains, and legumes can improve liver function and reduce the risk of liver disease. A study in *Nutrients* highlighted that plant-based diets are associated with lower liver enzyme levels and improved metabolic health.

Genetic Factors

Ongoing studies are investigating the genetic predisposition to liver diseases, which may help identify individuals at higher risk and tailor preventive strategies. Genetic factors can influence how individuals metabolize fats, respond to dietary changes, and develop liver conditions.

For instance, research has identified specific genetic variants associated with an increased risk of NAFLD. Understanding these genetic factors can lead to personalized dietary recommendations and interventions. Genetic testing may become a valuable tool in the future, allowing healthcare providers to identify individuals at risk and implement targeted lifestyle changes to prevent liver disease.

As research continues to evolve, innovative dietary approaches are being developed to support liver health. Here are some notable examples:

Personalized Nutrition

Advances in technology are enabling personalized nutrition plans based on individual genetic profiles, lifestyle factors, and health conditions. This tailored approach can optimize dietary choices for better liver health. For example, individuals with specific genetic markers may benefit from diets higher in omega-3 fatty acids or lower in saturated fats.

Personalized nutrition can also take into account an individual's microbiome composition, allowing for dietary recommendations that support gut health and, consequently, liver health. Companies are emerging that offer genetic testing and personalized meal plans, making it easier for individuals to make informed dietary choices.

Functional Foods

Research is identifying foods with specific health benefits for the liver, such as those rich in antioxidants, omega-3 fatty acids, and fiber. Incorporating these functional foods into the diet can enhance liver function and reduce the risk of liver disease.

For example, foods like turmeric, which contains the active compound curcumin, have been shown to have anti-inflammatory properties that may benefit liver health. Similarly, foods high in fiber, such as oats and legumes, can help regulate blood sugar levels and improve insulin sensitivity, both of which are important for liver health.

Plant-Based Diets: Studies are increasingly showing the benefits of plant-based diets in reducing liver fat and inflammation. These diets emphasize whole foods, fruits, vegetables, whole grains, and healthy fats. Research published in *The Journal of Nutrition* found that individuals following a plant-based diet had lower levels of liver fat and improved liver enzyme levels compared to those consuming a standard Western diet.

Plant-based diets are not only beneficial for liver health but also promote overall well-being. They are associated with lower risks of chronic diseases, including heart disease and diabetes, which are often linked to liver conditions.

The Role of Technology in Health Monitoring

Technology is playing a significant role in monitoring liver health and supporting lifestyle changes. Here are some innovations that are making a difference:

Wearable Devices

Fitness trackers and smartwatches can monitor physical activity, heart rate, and sleep patterns, providing valuable data to help individuals stay on track with their health goals. For example, devices like Fitbit or Apple Watch can track daily steps, encouraging users to meet their activity goals. Some devices also offer reminders to move, which can be particularly beneficial for those with sedentary lifestyles.

Health Apps

Mobile applications for tracking food intake, exercise, and health metrics can help individuals manage their liver health more effectively. Many apps, such as MyFitnessPal or Cronometer, allow users to log their meals and monitor their nutrient intake. These apps often provide educational resources and community support, making it easier for individuals to stay informed and motivated.

For instance, a user can log their meals and receive feedback on their macronutrient distribution, helping them make adjustments to align with their health goals. Some apps also offer features for tracking liver-specific health metrics, such as liver enzyme levels, which can be useful for individuals managing liver conditions.

Telehealth Services

Telehealth has become increasingly popular, allowing individuals to consult with healthcare professionals remotely. This can improve access to care and support for those managing liver health. Telehealth services enable patients to have regular check-ins with their healthcare providers without the need for in-person visits, making it easier to monitor progress and make necessary adjustments to treatment plans.

For example, a patient with NAFLD can schedule a virtual appointment with a registered dietitian to discuss their dietary changes and receive personalized guidance. This convenience can lead to better adherence to treatment plans and improved health outcomes.

Engaging with your community can provide valuable support and resources for managing liver health. Participating in health initiatives, support groups, and community programs can enhance your understanding of liver health and foster a sense of belonging.

Benefits of Participating in Health Initiatives

Community health initiatives often provide access to educational materials, workshops, and screenings that can enhance your understanding of liver health. These programs can empower individuals to take charge of their health and make informed decisions.

For example, local health organizations may offer workshops on nutrition, exercise, and lifestyle changes specifically tailored to liver health. Attending these workshops can provide valuable information and practical tips for managing your condition.

Finding Support Groups and Resources

Connecting with others who share similar health goals can foster a sense of belonging and motivation. Support groups can provide encouragement and accountability, making it easier to stay committed to your health journey.

Look for local health organizations, hospitals, or community centers that offer support groups focused on liver health or chronic disease management. Engaging with others who understand your challenges can be incredibly empowering and can help you feel less isolated in your journey.

Sharing your journey and knowledge with others can be incredibly rewarding. Consider the following:

- *Start a Blog or Social Media Account:* Document your health journey and share tips, recipes, and insights with others. This can inspire and motivate those who are facing similar challenges.

- *Volunteer*: Offer your time to local health organizations or community initiatives focused on liver health. Volunteering can provide a sense of purpose and connection.

- *Host Workshops*: If you feel comfortable, consider hosting workshops or informational sessions to educate others about liver health and healthy lifestyle choices.

Lifelong Learning and Adaptation

Importance of Staying Informed About Liver Health

Staying informed about liver health is crucial for making informed decisions and adapting your lifestyle as needed. Here are some ways to stay updated:

- *Follow Reputable Sources*: Subscribe to newsletters or follow organizations focused on liver health, such as the American Liver Foundation or the National Institute of Diabetes and Digestive and Kidney Diseases.

- *Attend Conferences and Webinars:* Participate in health conferences, webinars, or workshops to learn about the latest research and advancements in liver health.

- *Read Books and Articles*: Explore books, articles, and research papers related to liver health, nutrition, and lifestyle changes. This can deepen your understanding and provide new insights.

Adapting Dietary Choices as Needs Change

As you progress on your health journey, it's important to adapt your dietary choices based on your evolving needs. Consider the following:

- *Listen to Your Body*: Pay attention to how different foods affect your energy levels, digestion, and overall well-being. Adjust your diet accordingly to optimize your health.

- *Consult Healthcare Professionals*: Regularly check in with your healthcare provider or registered dietitian to discuss any changes in your health status and receive personalized guidance.

- *Be Open to Change*: Embrace the idea that your dietary needs may change over time. Stay flexible and willing to try new foods and approaches as you learn more about what works for you.

Embracing a Growth Mindset

Adopting a growth mindset can significantly impact your health journey. Here's how to cultivate this mindset:

- *View Challenges as Opportunities:* Instead of seeing setbacks as failures, view them as opportunities to learn and grow. Each challenge can provide valuable insights for your journey.

- *Celebrate Progress:* Acknowledge and celebrate your achievements, no matter how small. Recognizing your progress can boost your motivation and reinforce positive behaviors.

- *Stay Curious*: Approach your health journey with curiosity and a willingness to learn. This mindset can help you stay engaged and motivated as you explore new strategies for improving your liver health.

As we look to the future of liver health, it's clear that ongoing education, community engagement, and a commitment to lifelong learning are essential components of your health journey. In the conclusion, we will reflect on the key takeaways from this book and emphasize the importance of taking control of your liver health for a brighter, healthier future.

Conclusion

As we reach the end of this journey together, it's important to reflect on the transformative power of managing fatty liver disease through diet and lifestyle changes. The path to better liver health is not just about making dietary adjustments; it's about embracing a holistic approach that encompasses physical activity, stress management, and community support. Each step you take toward healthier choices is a step toward reclaiming your vitality and well-being.

Throughout this book, we have explored the essential components of managing fatty liver disease effectively. We began by understanding the condition itself and the critical role that diet plays in liver health. We discussed the importance of incorporating nutrient-dense foods, creating a sustainable meal plan, and overcoming challenges related to cravings and social situations. We also highlighted the significance of physical activity, stress management, and building a supportive community. Finally, we emphasized the need for ongoing monitoring of your progress and adapting your strategies as your needs change.

By implementing the strategies and recipes provided, you can take control of your liver health and make meaningful changes that positively impact your life.

Now is the time to take the first step toward better liver health. By incorporating what you have learned in this book; the recipes, meal planning techniques, and overall liver health management strategies into your daily routine. Remember, every small change counts, and consistency is key. Whether it's swapping out a sugary snack for a piece of fruit or committing to a daily walk, each decision you make brings you closer to your health goals.

Managing fatty liver disease is a journey that requires patience, dedication, and self-compassion. It's important to remember that setbacks may occur, but they do not define your progress. Embrace the process, celebrate your victories, and seek support when needed. With the right mindset and resources, you can navigate this journey with confidence and resilience.

As you move forward, know that you have the power to create a healthier, more fulfilling life. Your liver health is within your control, and by making informed choices, you can pave the way for a brighter future. Here's to your health and the exciting journey ahead!

Your Feedback Means A Lot!

Dear Reader,

Thank you for taking the time to explore "The Essential Fatty Liver Diet Guide: Recipes and Tips for Liver Health." Your journey toward better liver health is important, and I hope this book has provided you with valuable insights, practical strategies, and delicious recipes to support your health goals.

As you continue on your path to wellness, I would be incredibly grateful if you could take a moment to share your thoughts about the book by leaving a review on Amazon. Your feedback not only helps me improve future editions but also assists other readers in finding the resources they need to manage their liver health effectively.

You may leave a review by simply typing this link on your computer's browser: ***https://go.binnovatedigital.com/FLDG***

Alternatively, you may scan this QR code using your phone's camera:

Thank you very much!

Sincerest Regards,

Dorothy

Reference

American Liver Foundation
> Title: Fatty Liver Disease Overview
> Link: https://www.liverfoundation.org

National Institute of Diabetes and Digestive and Kidney Diseases
> Title: Non-Alcoholic Fatty Liver Disease
> Link: https://www.niddk.nih.gov

U.S. Department of Agriculture
> Title: Dietary Guidelines for Americans
> Link: https://www.dietaryguidelines.gov

Mayo Clinic
> Title: Nonalcoholic Fatty Liver Disease
> Link: https://www.mayoclinic.org/diseases-conditions/nonalcoholic-fatty-liver-disease/symptoms-causes/syc-20347466

Cleveland Clinic
> Title: Fatty Liver Disease: Symptoms, Causes, and Treatment
> Link: https://my.clevelandclinic.org/health/diseases/21782-fatty-liver-disease

Harvard Health Publishing
> Title: The Liver: A Vital Organ
> Link: https://www.health.harvard.edu/diseases-and-conditions/the-liver-a-vital-organ

World Health Organization
> Title: Healthy Diet
> Link: https://www.who.int/news-room/fact-sheets/detail/healthy-diet

National Institute of Health
> Title: The Role of Nutrition in Liver Disease
> Link: https://www.ncbi.nlm.nih.gov/pmc/articles/PMC6466100/

American Association for the Study of Liver Diseases
> Title: AASLD Practice Guidelines: Nonalcoholic Fatty Liver Disease
> Link: https://www.aasld.org/sites/default/files/2020-09/NAFLD%20Guideline%20Summary%20for%20Patients.pdf

Cleveland Clinic
> Title: 10 Tips for a Healthy Liver
> Link: https://health.clevelandclinic.org/10-tips-for-a-healthy-liver/

Index

The topics are indexed according to the chapter(s) they appear in this book.

www.ingramcontent.com/pod-product-compliance
Lightning Source LLC
Chambersburg PA
CBHW060245030426
42335CB00014B/1598